GROW & KNOW

Written by Marni Sommer, Margaret Schmitt,
Christine Hagstrom and Caitlin Gruer

Stories written by girls across the USA

Book design & illustration
by Emily Scheffler; minuscule studio

For more information, please visit www.GrowandKnow.org

In honor of Sid Lerner, a champion for
empowering young people around the world to
learn about their growing bodies.

FOREWORD:

This book was developed through participatory research with young people across the USA. Adolescents were asked to share the questions they wanted answered, the information they need, and to write stories about their first menstrual period experience; a selection of which are included in this book.

We also talked with adults in young people's lives, such as teachers, social workers, healthcare workers, and religious leaders, so we would understand what they worry about and feel young people should learn. This all shapes the book content, which also incorporates factual content from child health and development literature.

Our hope is that young people ages 9-14 read this book and feel more confident and knowledgeable about their changing bodies, and that families, teachers, youth leaders and others introduce these books to the young people in their lives reaching and going through puberty.

TABLE OF CONTENTS

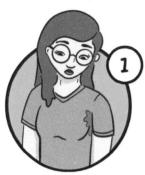

1 BODY CHANGES!

Introduction 9
Hormones + Emotions 11
Breast Growth 14
Pimples + Body Smells 16
Hair + Discharge 17

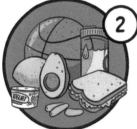

2 CARING FOR YOUR BODY

Growing + Eating 20
Exercise + Sleep 22

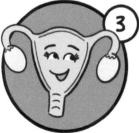

3 WHAT'S A PERIOD ALL ABOUT?

All About Periods 26
Leaks + Blood 28
PMS 30
Cramps 31

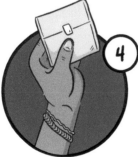

4 CARING FOR YOUR PERIOD

Period Products 36
Tracking Your Period 42

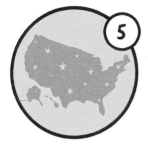

5 MY FIRST PERIOD: STORIES FROM REAL GIRLS

My Surprise Summer with Dad 46
An Unexpected Summer Visitor 51
A New Type of Math Class Problem 58
My Purple Pants Panic 64
Aunt Sara to the Rescue! 68
My Fourth Grade Shock 72
The Case of the Slowpoke Period 76
Grandma Saves the Day 80

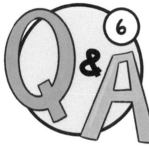

6 ALL THE FACTS!

Period Myth Busters 88
Questions + Answers 90

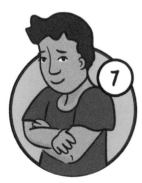

7 WHAT ABOUT BOYS?

What's Going on in HIS Body? 98

8 GLOSSARY

. . . . 103

Pay attention to <u>underlined purple words</u> in the book! You can find those words in the glossary.

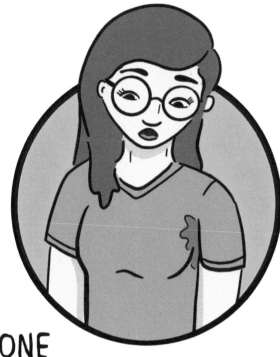

CHAPTER ONE
BODY CHANGES!

WHAT IS HAPPENING TO MY BODY?

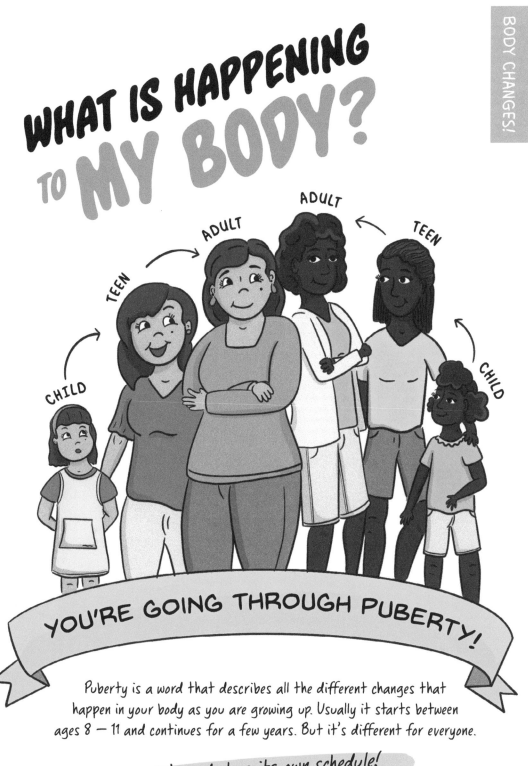

ADULT

ADULT

TEEN

TEEN

CHILD

CHILD

YOU'RE GOING THROUGH PUBERTY!

Puberty is a word that describes all the different changes that happen in your body as you are growing up. Usually it starts between ages 8 — 11 and continues for a few years. But it's different for everyone.

Everyone's body has its own schedule!

SOME OF THESE CHANGES YOU CAN SEE:

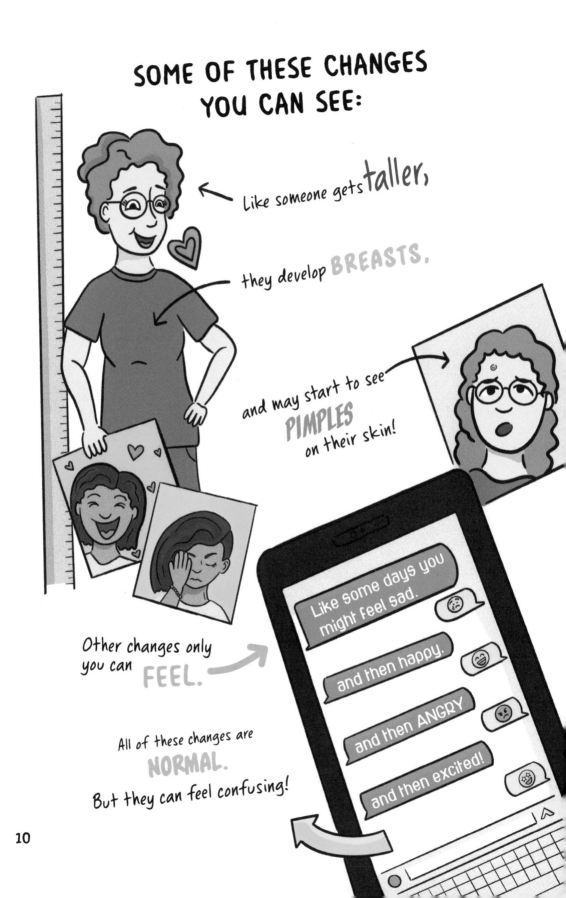

Like someone gets taller,

they develop BREASTS,

and may start to see PIMPLES on their skin!

Other changes only you can FEEL.

All of these changes are NORMAL.
But they can feel confusing!

Like some days you might feel sad.

and then happy.

and then ANGRY

and then excited!

HORMONES

HORMONES ARE CHEMICALS THAT CHANGE A GIRL'S BODY INTO A YOUNG WOMAN'S BODY.

They also change a boy's body into a young man's body. But we'll talk about that later! For girls, puberty usually lasts around 6 years.

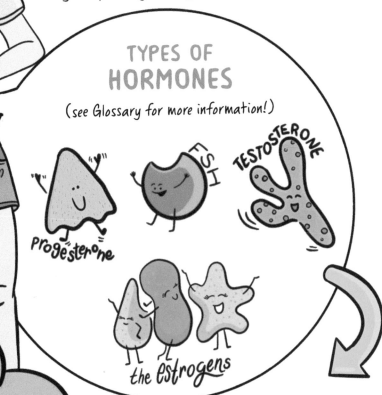

TYPES OF HORMONES

(see Glossary for more information!)

"♀" Progesterone

FSH

TESTOSTERONE

the Estrogens

REMEMBER!

Each person has a different body. Don't worry if your body is showing changes faster or slower than your friends!

DIFFERENT HORMONES HAVE DIFFERENT JOBS IN YOUR BODY.

Estrogen helps trigger some of the physical changes in your body you can see- like growing breasts and hair!

Progesterone and Testosterone do things like help regulate your menstrual cycle every month.

11

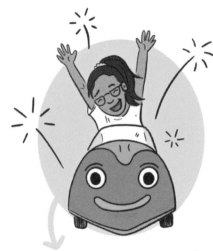

SO MANY BIG EMOTIONS!

Hormones do more than just make changes in your body- they can also affect your mood and emotions.

You might find that you're feeling more sensitive than you used to- like little things make you sad or upset more quickly or easily.

You might also begin to feel more self-conscious, worried, and stressed about all the big changes going on in your life and your body.

IT'S NORMAL TO HAVE "BIG FEELINGS."

ON TOP OF THE WORLD!

THE BLUES

SAD & LONELY
When I'm feeling sad, I like to pet my cat or listen to my favorite music.

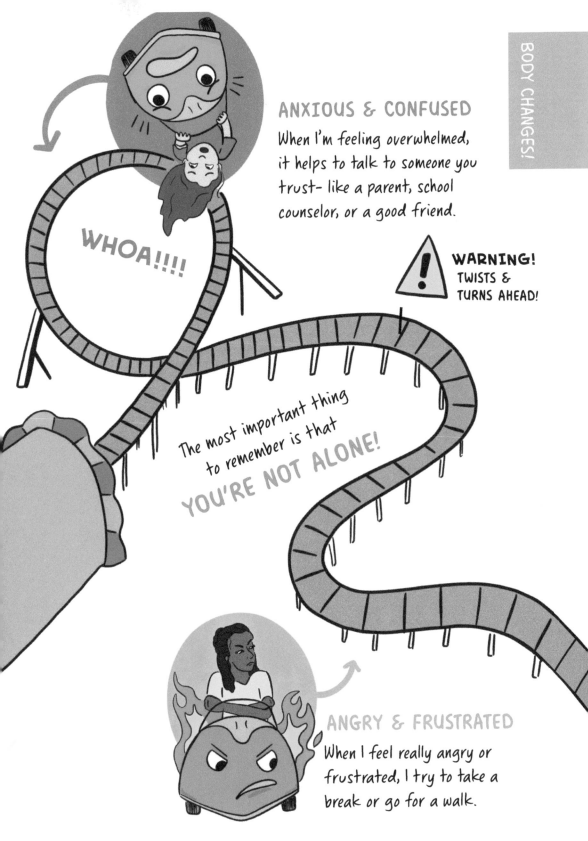

ANXIOUS & CONFUSED

When I'm feeling overwhelmed, it helps to talk to someone you trust- like a parent, school counselor, or a good friend.

WHOA!!!!

WARNING!
TWISTS & TURNS AHEAD!

The most important thing to remember is that YOU'RE NOT ALONE!

ANGRY & FRUSTRATED

When I feel really angry or frustrated, I try to take a break or go for a walk.

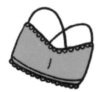

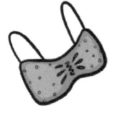

HOW WILL YOUR BREASTS CHANGE?

Each person's breasts will grow a little differently. But feel proud of your own breast changes! They are special to you. Don't worry if your breasts are growing slower or faster than your friends. Some people start to wear bras when their breasts develop, but it's up to you to decide what makes you most comfortable!

Also, sometimes the area around the breasts may feel a little sore. It's nothing to worry about! It's just a part of growing.

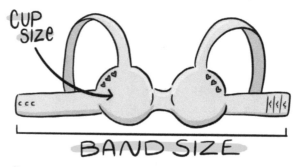

THE ABCs OF BRA SIZES!!

There are two parts to a bra's size:
the CHEST or BAND SIZE and the CUP SIZE.

CUP SIZE

BAND SIZE

The "cup" is the part that holds your breasts. They come in letter sizes like AA, A, B, C, D...etc. The "band" is the part that runs across your chest and around your back. Chest or band size is represented by a number like 34, 36, 38...and so on.

5 STAGES OF
BREAST GROWTH
AND OTHER BODY CHANGES

STAGE 1:
No breast development (yet!)

STAGE 2:
Breasts begin to "bud"

STAGE 3:
Breasts get bigger and fuller

STAGE 4:
The nipple becomes distinct from the aureola

STAGE 5:
Breasts are fully mature

OTHER BODY CHANGES DURING THESE STAGES:

Internal hormonal changes are happening

Pubic hair growth, body odors, and growth spurt

Pubic hair darkens and vaginal discharge begins

Menstruation begins (Your first period!)

Pubic hair extends to inner thighs and height growth stops

15

PIMPLES!? (ALSO KNOWN AS ACNE)

Your body will also start to produce more oil. On your face, this oil can mix with bacteria and dead skin cells. Wash your face with soap and water, and try not to touch your face. Both help to keep the pimples away!

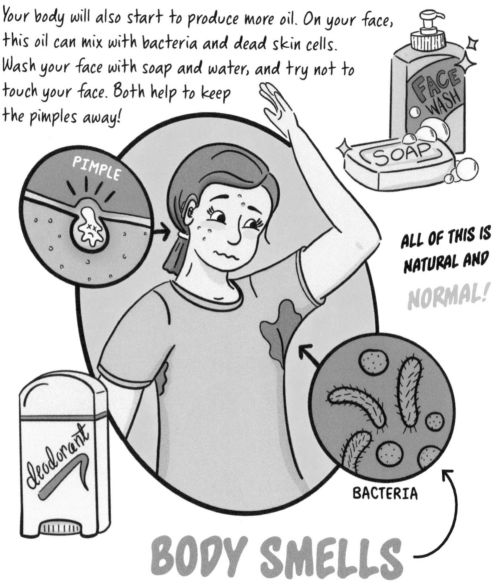

PIMPLE

ALL OF THIS IS NATURAL AND NORMAL!

deodorant

BACTERIA

BODY SMELLS

You may notice some new stronger smells as your body starts to sweat more, including a change in smell under your arms on hotter days. When you sweat, it mixes with bacteria and can smell a bit more!

Taking regular baths or showers and using deodorant (or anti-perspirant) under your arms can help you to manage the smell!

HAIR?!
SO MANY CHANGES!

First you might see "pubic hair" growing between your hip bones. It is often soft and straight at the beginning, then it usually becomes curly.

You might see more hair start to grow on your arms, in your armpits or even on your face. It is all normal!

Some girls like to keep the hair, and some girls like to remove it. Either way is ok, but it's always a good idea to ask an older person who you trust for advice before removing it.

The hair on your head may also start to feel oily.

PUBIC AREA

ALL OF THIS IS NORMAL!

DISCHARGE

You may start to see some discharge on your underwear. Sometimes the discharge is clear, white or an off-white color.

DON'T BE WORRIED!

This is a normal and healthy sign that you are growing inside.

clear

white

off-white

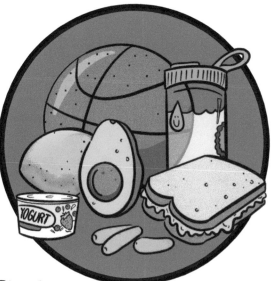

CHAPTER TWO

CARING FOR YOUR BODY!

AND YOU GROW!

GROWTH SPURTS

These are the years when you will get taller and taller. Some girls experience growth spurts much earlier than boys and other girls their age.

WEIGHT GAIN

You will start to grow hips, with the sides of your body growing **ROUNDER** and **FULLER.**

Growing taller and gaining weight are more signs that you are becoming a young adult!

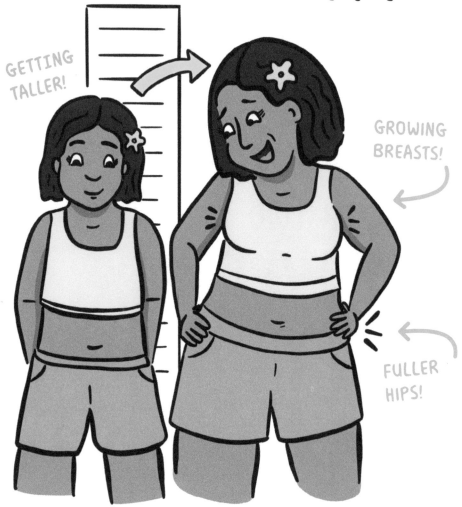

GETTING TALLER!

GROWING BREASTS!

FULLER HIPS!

ALL THIS GROWTH CAN MAKE YOU FEEL

HUNGRIER,

Eating to fill your body's growing needs is important, but it's also important to eat foods that are good for your body. You need healthy food that will help your body and brain grow.

It's important to eat the right amount for your body. Not too much or too little!

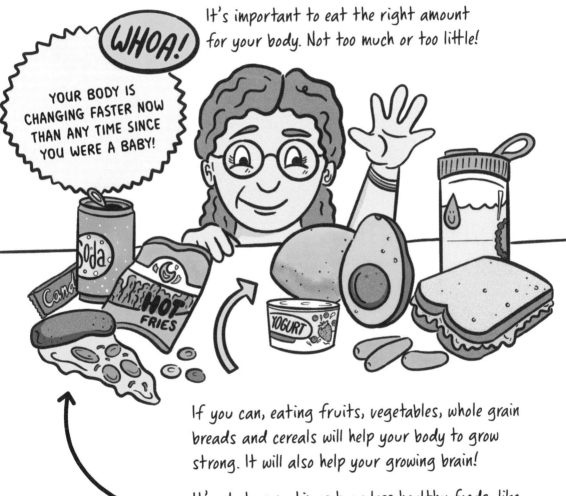

WHOA!

YOUR BODY IS CHANGING FASTER NOW THAN ANY TIME SINCE YOU WERE A BABY!

If you can, eating fruits, vegetables, whole grain breads and cereals will help your body to grow strong. It will also help your growing brain!

It's ok to sometimes have less healthy foods, like candy or sugary soda or fried foods. Just try to eat them in small amounts.

21

EXERCISE

YOUR BODY NEEDS EXERCISE TO STAY HEALTHY AND GROW!

It helps your muscles and bones grow, and it is also good for your mood! Exercising regularly may reduce stress, can create feelings of happiness, and help you to feel strong and confident in your body.

STAIRS

Try to take the stairs instead of the elevator!

SLEEP

Getting enough sleep is also so important! Your body and brain are doing SO much growing during these years.

Scientists recommend **8 TO 11** hours per night.

PRO TIP!
Avoid screens before bedtime to help you sleep better.

Try to go to bed at the same time each night. Regular sleeping hours will improve the quality of your rest!

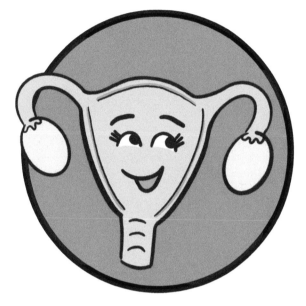

CHAPTER THREE

WHAT'S A PERIOD ALL ABOUT?

ALL ABOUT PERIODS!

A "period" is a part of something called your menstrual cycle. It happens to girls and women about once a month and you'll bleed a little bit from your vagina. It usually lasts 3-7 days. Don't worry-it's not because you're hurt!

IT'S A NATURAL AND NORMAL PROCESS THAT ALL GIRLS AND WOMEN GO THROUGH!

There's an organ in your body called the uterus where a woman's body prepares itself to have a baby.

UTERUS

OVARIES

VAGINA

During your cycle, your uterus builds up a cushy lining on the inside and then sheds it. This is where the blood you'll see comes from.

WHY IS IT CALLED A CYCLE?

Your menstrual cycle has four main stages that repeat over and over- just like a circle. A regular cycle happens on average every 21-35 days, but some girls have shorter cycles and some girls have longer ones! A cycle can also vary. So, don't worry if your period comes after 29 days one month, and after 33 days the next month.

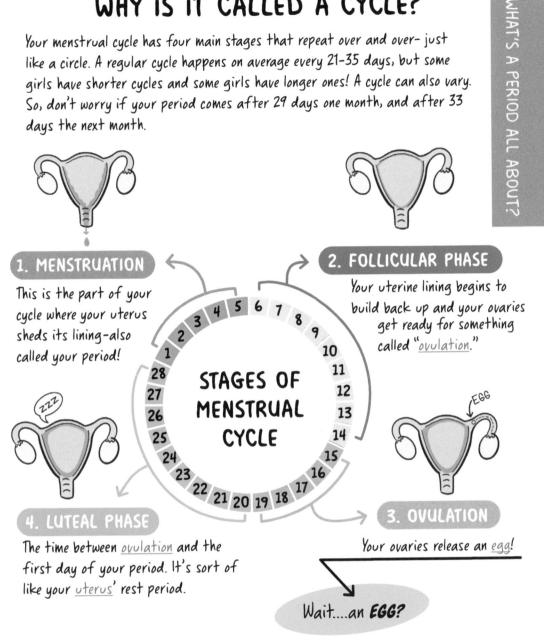

1. MENSTRUATION

This is the part of your cycle where your uterus sheds its lining-also called your period!

2. FOLLICULAR PHASE

Your uterine lining begins to build back up and your ovaries get ready for something called "_ovulation_."

STAGES OF MENSTRUAL CYCLE

EGG

4. LUTEAL PHASE

The time between _ovulation_ and the first day of your period. It's sort of like your _uterus'_ rest period.

3. OVULATION

Your ovaries release an _egg_!

Wait....an **EGG?**

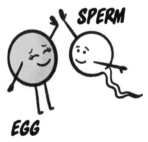

SPERM

EGG

WHAT ARE EGGS AND SPERM??

You won't be able to see it, but inside your growing body, you have "_eggs_" that are developing. And inside a boy's body, there is something called "sperm" that are developing. One day, when you are much older, these eggs and sperm together are what help to make a baby.

27

SO...HOW MUCH BLOOD WILL THERE BE?

There is no right "amount." On the first day or two it is usually a heavier blood flow. And then it slows. Usually it's about the amount of two to three tablespoons in total for your whole period. If you think you are bleeding more than this, talk to a parent or caregiver for advice.

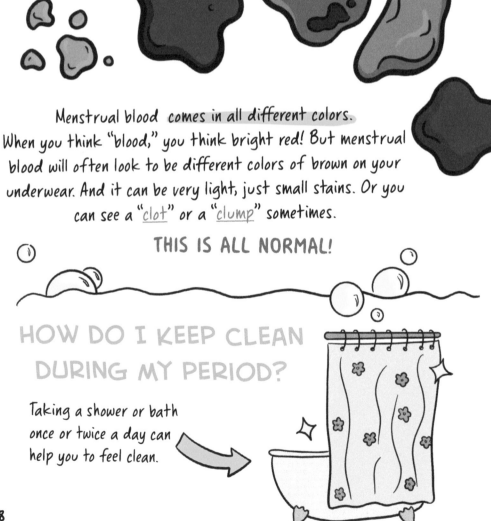

1 TABLESPOON

WHAT DOES PERIOD BLOOD LOOK LIKE?

Menstrual blood comes in all different colors. When you think "blood," you think bright red! But menstrual blood will often look to be different colors of brown on your underwear. And it can be very light, just small stains. Or you can see a "clot" or a "clump" sometimes.

THIS IS ALL NORMAL!

HOW DO I KEEP CLEAN DURING MY PERIOD?

Taking a shower or bath once or twice a day can help you to feel clean.

WHAT ABOUT
LEAKS?

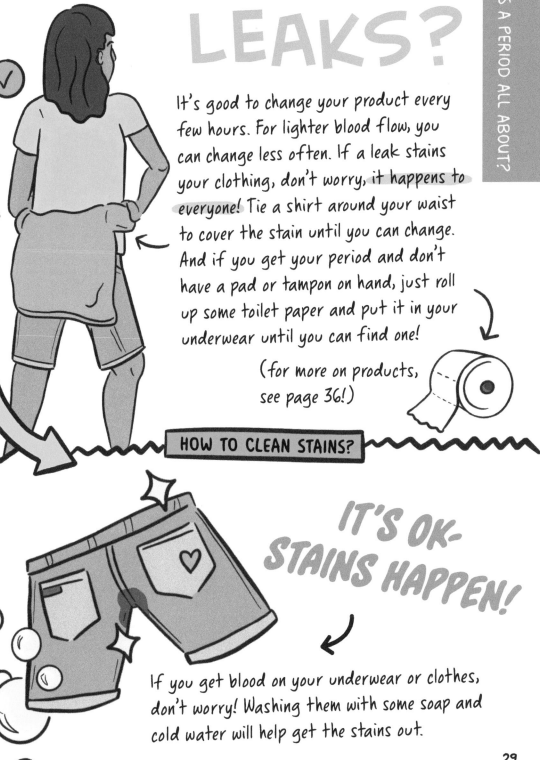

It's good to change your product every few hours. For lighter blood flow, you can change less often. If a leak stains your clothing, don't worry, it happens to everyone! Tie a shirt around your waist to cover the stain until you can change. And if you get your period and don't have a pad or tampon on hand, just roll up some toilet paper and put it in your underwear until you can find one!

(for more on products, see page 36!)

HOW TO CLEAN STAINS?

IT'S OK- STAINS HAPPEN!

If you get blood on your underwear or clothes, don't worry! Washing them with some soap and cold water will help get the stains out.

29

PMS

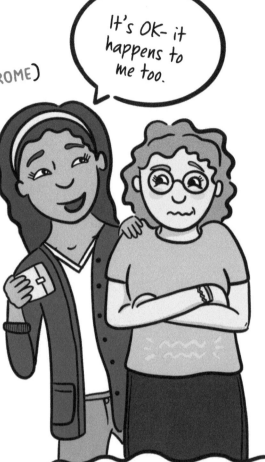

It's OK- it happens to me too.

It's not a disease or anything bad. Just a natural result of your body's hormones!

PMS refers to all the different things that you can feel before you get your period.

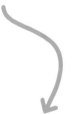

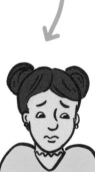

Some girls feel like their breasts are swollen or sore for a few days.

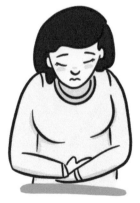

Other girls will feel like their stomach is full or **BLOATED.**

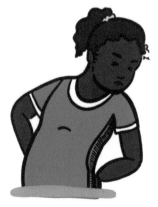

Some will also feel pain in their lower back.

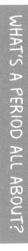

PMS CAN ALSO MAKE YOU FEEL

EMOTIONAL

These symptoms will go away soon after your period arrives. If you are worried about PMS, talk to an adult about it.

ALL THESE THINGS ARE

NORMAL!

BUT WHAT ABOUT THOSE THINGS CALLED

CRAMPS?

When your <u>uterus</u> contracts (or squeezes!) to push out the tissue that you see as "menstrual blood," the feeling of the muscles squeezing is called "cramps." For some girls this can be very painful, while others may not feel it at all.

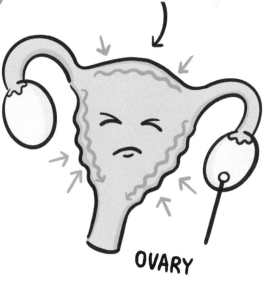

UTERUS

OVARY

HOW DO YOU MANAGE CRAMPS?

It's always good to ask someone you trust for advice on cramps. Some people like to take pain medicine, like ibuprofen (but make sure to get this from an adult!).

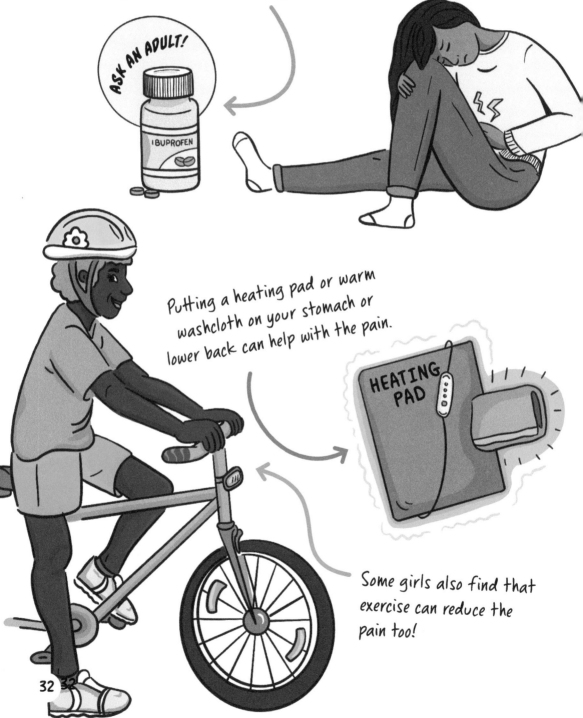

ASK AN ADULT!

IBUPROFEN

Putting a heating pad or warm washcloth on your stomach or lower back can help with the pain.

HEATING PAD

Some girls also find that exercise can reduce the pain too!

WHAT DO GIRLS ALL OVER AMERICA CALL THEIR PERIODS?

Getting your period is something to be proud of! It is an important sign that your body is growing up.

CALLING YOUR PERIOD BY ITS REAL NAME – A PERIOD! – IS GREAT!

But some girls like to give fun nicknames to their periods. Girls across the USA shared all different names for their periods that they use with friends!

HELLO MY NAME IS:

T.O.M.
(TIME OF MONTH)

half moon
La media luna

AUNT FLO

JUST PLAIN OLD
PERIOD.

THE RED DOT

SHARK WEEK!

"MONTHLIES"
TO: YOU
SPECIAL DELIVERY!

THE RED SEA

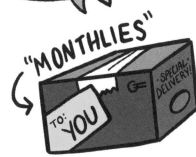
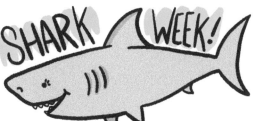
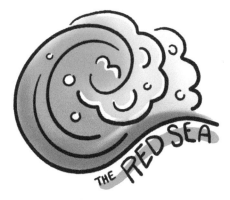
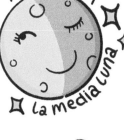

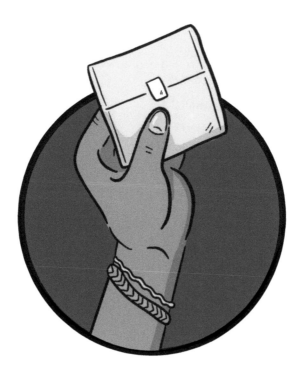

CHAPTER FOUR
CARING FOR YOUR PERIOD

SO MANY PERIOD PRODUCTS!

It can be confusing knowing what product to use! How do you know what type to choose? The next section has some basic facts about the most common types. But remember, there is no right or wrong answer. It's about what's most comfortable for you!

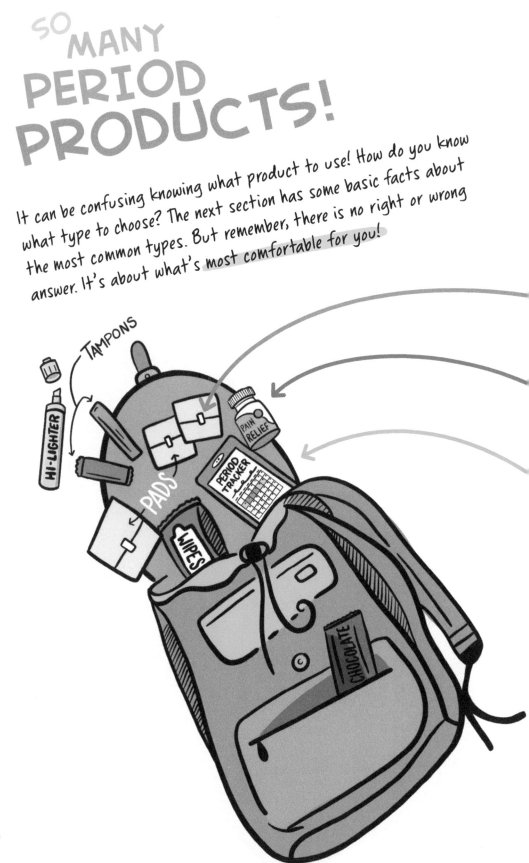

PRO TIPS:
WHAT'S IN YOUR BAG?

Your period can be irregular! When a girl starts menstruating, her period may not come as regularly for the first year or two. That's normal! But it does mean you need to be prepared. Here are some tips from a few girls about what they like to do:

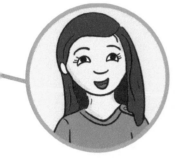

"I always carry an extra product—or two—just in case! You never know when you (or a friend!) might need one. I like to use pads, so I keep a couple extra in one of my backpack's pockets."

(more about products- page 38!)

"I often get cramps when I'm on my period. Sometimes I go lay down on a cot in the nurse's office if the cramps are really bad. (They might also have extra products in case you forget!) I also keep my favorite snack in my backpack for when I'm feeling down."

(more about cramps- page 31!)

"My period isn't 'regular' yet, but tracking my cycle on a calendar helps me estimate when it will start!"

(more about tracking- page 42!)

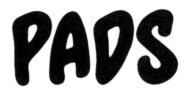

PADS

PANTY LINER OR PAD?

A pad is thicker and more absorbent, so it can hold more liquid (blood) than a panty liner. Panty liners can be worn on light bleeding days, or when wearing a tampon to give extra protection.

THIN OR MEDIUM OR THICK?
WINGS OR NO WINGS?

For lighter flow days, you can wear a thin pad. For heavier flow days, you can wear a medium or thick pad. For sleeping, you might prefer a thicker overnight pad.

Some girls prefer pads with wings, which wrap around the bottom of your underwear, but it is completely up to you!

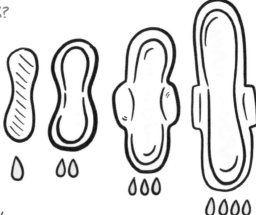

HOW LONG SHOULD YOU WEAR IT?

On average, for 2-3 hours. When your period is lighter, change every 6-8 hours. Some people may have a heavier period flow and need to change more often.

WHAT ABOUT DISPOSAL?

Wrap pads in tissue, a product wrapper or toilet paper and put into the trash can. Don't try to flush a pad down the toilet because it might get clogged.

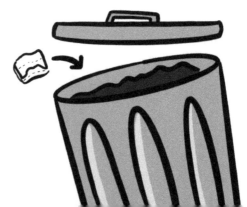

HOW TO PUT ON A PAD

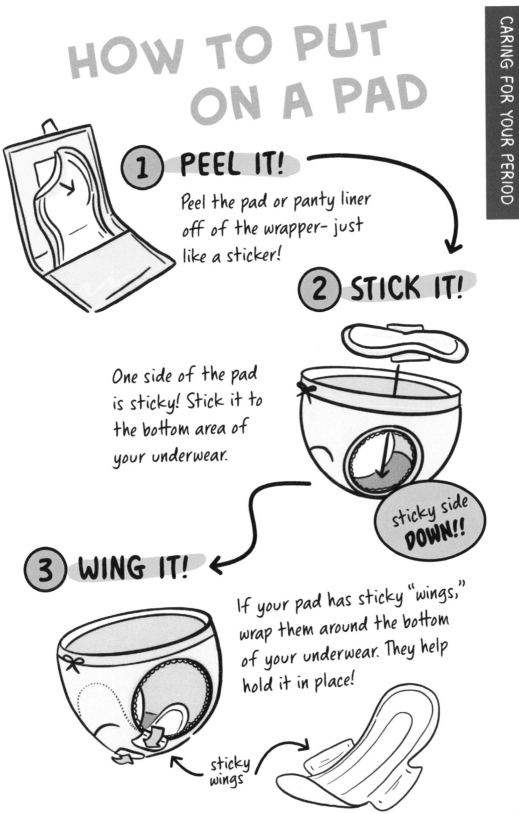

1 PEEL IT!

Peel the pad or panty liner off of the wrapper— just like a sticker!

2 STICK IT!

One side of the pad is sticky! Stick it to the bottom area of your underwear.

sticky side **DOWN!!**

3 WING IT!

If your pad has sticky "wings," wrap them around the bottom of your underwear. They help hold it in place!

sticky wings

39

TAMPONS

LIGHT OR REGULAR OR SUPER?

You can try them all and see which is most comfortable! Most girls start with "light." If your blood flow is very heavy, you might want to change to the regular or super sizes.

APPLICATOR OR NO APPLICATOR?

This is up to you! You can try both and see which you like best. (For more about tampons, see page 89!)

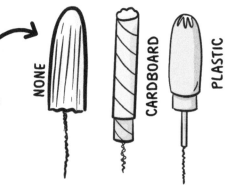

NONE **CARDBOARD** **PLASTIC**

HOW LONG SHOULD YOU WEAR IT?

On average, for 2-3 hours. When your period is lighter, change every 6-8 hours. Some people may have a heavier period flow and need to change more often. It's best not to wear one for longer than 8 hours though.

NEVER FLUSH YOUR PRODUCTS!

WHAT ABOUT DISPOSAL?

The same as pads! Wrap them in tissue, a product wrapper or toilet paper and put into the trash can. Remember— NEVER flush them down the toilet!

PERIOD UNDERWEAR

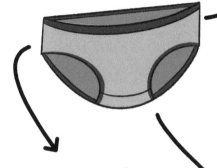

WHAT ARE THEY?

Period underwear is special underwear that has an absorbent material in it to soak up blood. You can wash and reuse them!

WHAT SIZE?

The same size as your other underwear! They come in different fits and styles — so select one you find most comfortable!

WHAT THICKNESS?

Up to you! If you have heavier blood flow, try thicker options.

HOW LONG SHOULD YOU WEAR THEM?

Depends on your blood flow! Change once or twice a day. To wash them, read the instructions provided as some can go directly into a washing machine and others should be washed by hand.

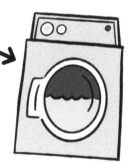

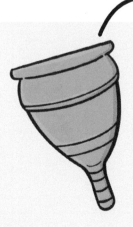

MENSTRUAL CUPS

Some people like to use menstrual cups. You can use a cup over and over. Similar to tampons, cups are inserted into the vagina. Most cups are reusable. Ask an adult or look at the product box for more information.

41

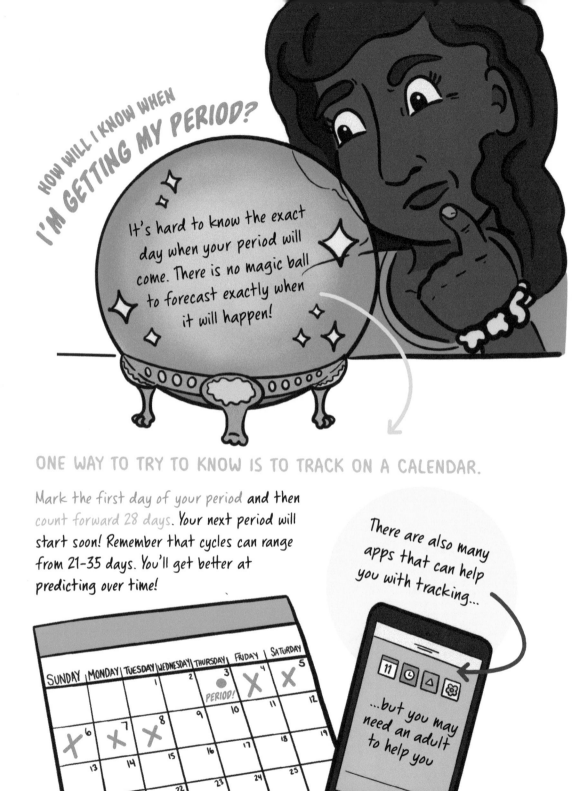

HOW WILL I KNOW WHEN I'M GETTING MY PERIOD?

It's hard to know the exact day when your period will come. There is no magic ball to forecast exactly when it will happen!

ONE WAY TO TRY TO KNOW IS TO TRACK ON A CALENDAR.

Mark the first day of your period and then count forward 28 days. Your next period will start soon! Remember that cycles can range from 21-35 days. You'll get better at predicting over time!

There are also many apps that can help you with tracking...

...but you may need an adult to help you

HAVE MORE
QUESTIONS?

That's totally OK! This is a confusing time. Talk to someone who you trust! It's a good idea to talk to someone who has been having their period for years like your mother, older sister, aunt, teacher, cousin, older friend, or school nurse. They will have lots of good advice for you!

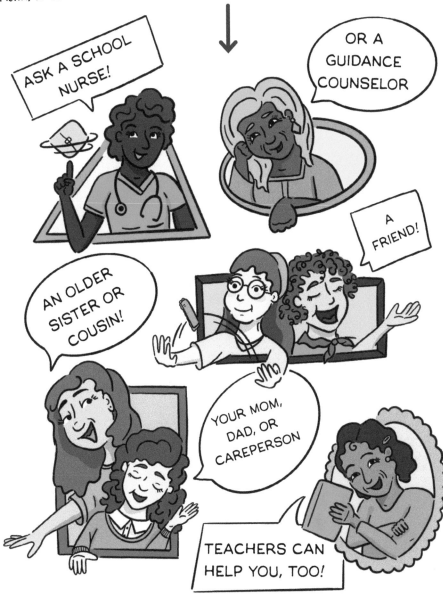

ASK A SCHOOL NURSE!

OR A GUIDANCE COUNSELOR

A FRIEND!

AN OLDER SISTER OR COUSIN!

YOUR MOM, DAD, OR CAREPERSON

TEACHERS CAN HELP YOU, TOO!

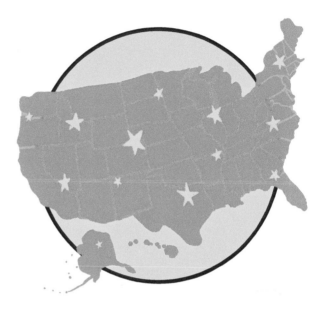

CHAPTER FIVE

MY FIRST PERIOD: STORIES FROM REAL GIRLS

The following section has a selection of stories from girls all across the USA about their first period! Just like every girl is unique, every person's experience is a little different- and yours will be too! Just remember that you're not alone- everyone goes through puberty!

STORY 1: MY SURPRISE SUMMER WITH DAD

I got my first period when I was 12 years old.

I was visiting my dad in Seattle for the summer, so I had no immediate menstruating relatives close to me.

My doctor had told me that I might get my period soon, but I wasn't that worried.

MOM

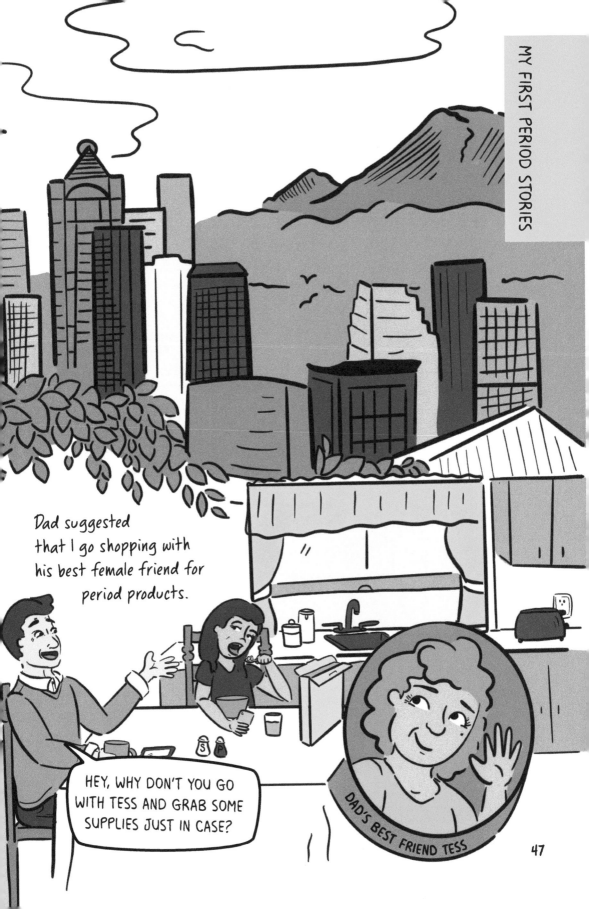

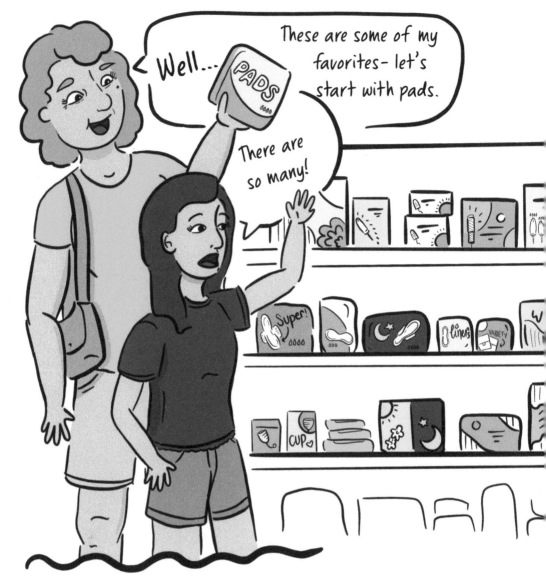

It's a good thing I did because about a week later, I went to the bathroom and noticed blood in my underwear!

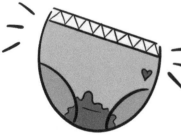

I knew what a period was and even what to expect, but you can never truly prepare for your first period. I started to cry because I was scared.

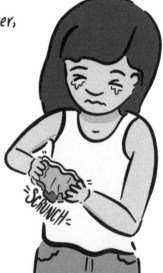

It's like a big sticker!

SO...I TOOK A DEEP BREATH AND CALLED MY MOM.

She made me feel a lot better and taught me how to put on a pad over the phone.

Thankfully, my dad was super supportive and took me out to buy all the foods I was craving. My dad and I have always had a close relationship, so I was never afraid to tell him about anything, including my period.

I remember texting him and telling him I felt like a leaky faucet because when I got up to get another pad, I leaked onto the bathroom floor.

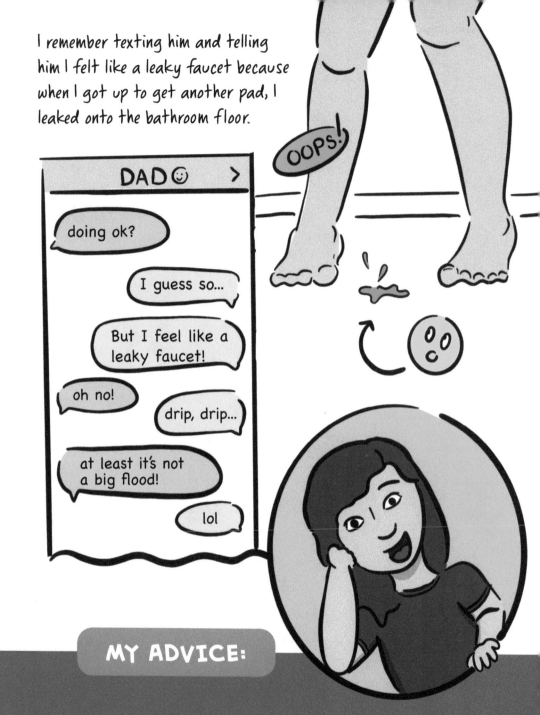

OOPS!

DAD☺ ›

doing ok?

I guess so...

But I feel like a leaky faucet!

oh no!

drip, drip...

at least it's not a big flood!

lol

MY ADVICE:

I would tell young people who are newly menstruating that it's ok to feel scared when you get your first period, and that periods are something you shouldn't be ashamed of.

THE END!

STORY 2: AN UNEXPECTED SUMMER VISITOR

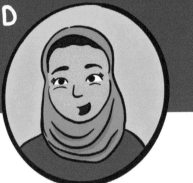

I got my period on August 9th 2016, when I was 13.

My cousins were visiting for the summer vacation, so we decided to go to the park.

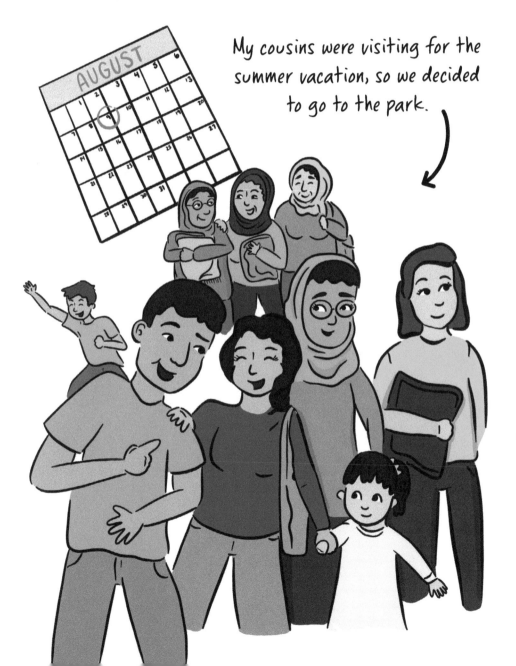

I went with my sisters, my cousins, my aunts and my mom. I was wearing grey sweats and brought a sweater in case it got chilly.

LATER ON...

As I was playing, I suddenly noticed a stain on my sweats. I thought that it was mud, so I brushed it off and continued to play.

There was a movie showing in the park that evening, so we decided to stay and watch.

As we were leaving, my mom noticed the stain from before and realized I got my period. She quickly tied my sweater around my waist, and we rushed home. I was really confused as to what was happening and felt scared.

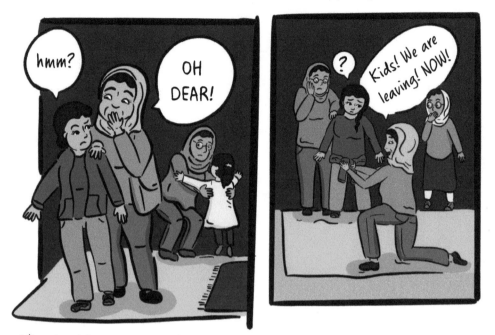

When I got home, my mom told me to go straight to the bathroom, and when I pulled down my underpants I saw I was bleeding. I was really confused...

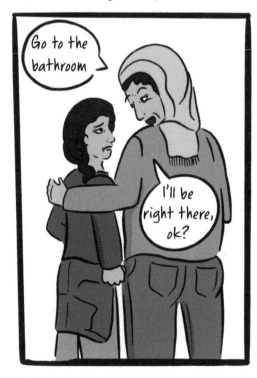

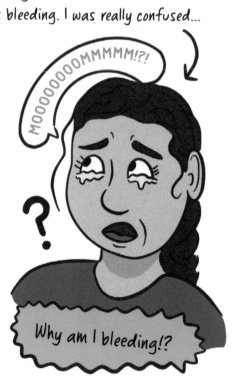

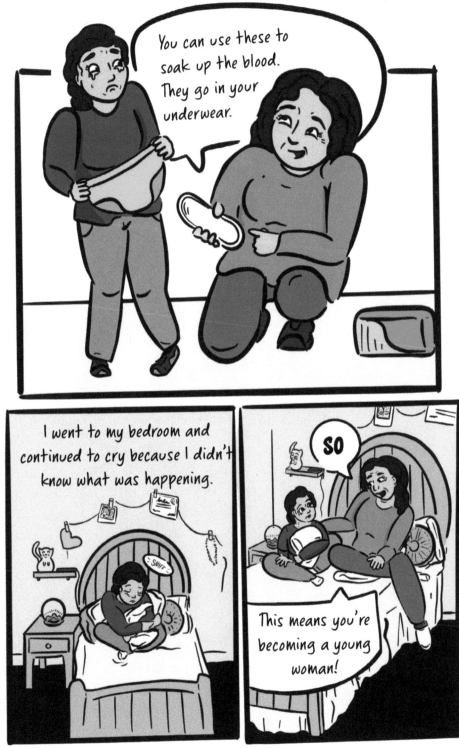

Although my mom explained things to me, she didn't get into much detail. Afterwards I went on the internet to try to learn more.

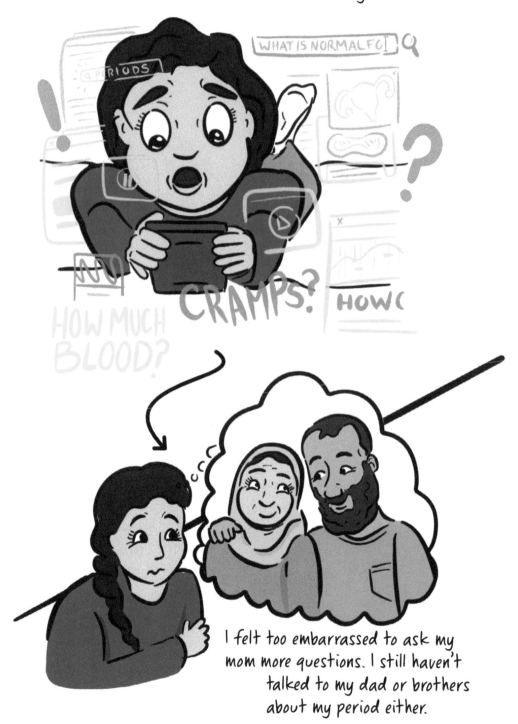

I felt too embarrassed to ask my mom more questions. I still haven't talked to my dad or brothers about my period either.

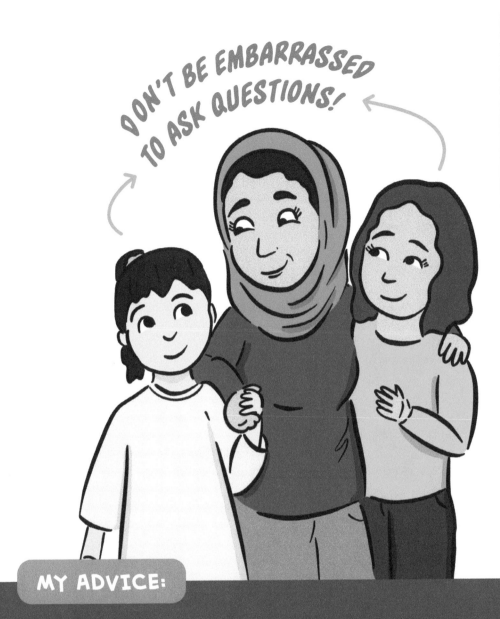

DON'T BE EMBARRASSED TO ASK QUESTIONS!

MY ADVICE:

I want my sisters to know they can ask me or others they trust any questions they may have about periods. I was not comfortable and relied on the internet, which didn't always answer my questions and was sometimes really overwhelming!

THE END!

57

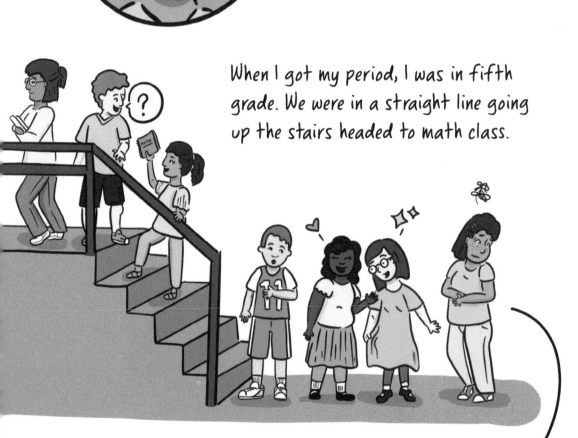

When I got my period, I was in fifth
grade. We were in a straight line going
up the stairs headed to math class.

As we went up, I started to feel uncomfortable,
and my back started to hurt.

As we walked inside our classroom, I started to
feel stomach pains and aching.

After trying to ignore the pain, I decided to raise my hand to use the bathroom...

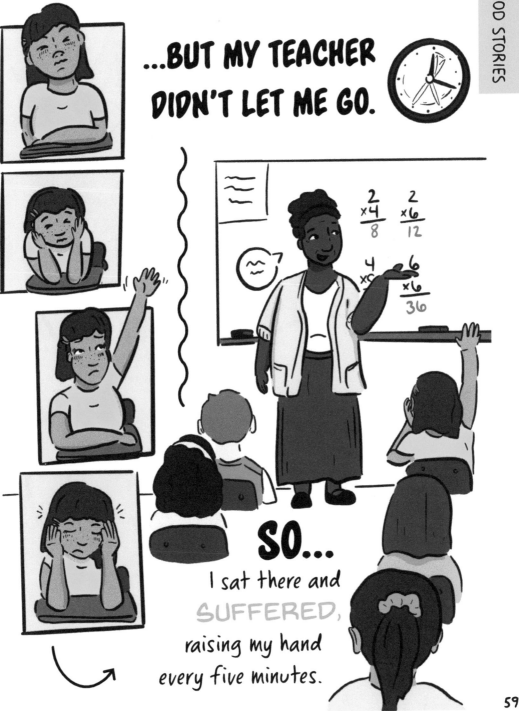

...BUT MY TEACHER DIDN'T LET ME GO.

SO...

I sat there and SUFFERED, raising my hand every five minutes.

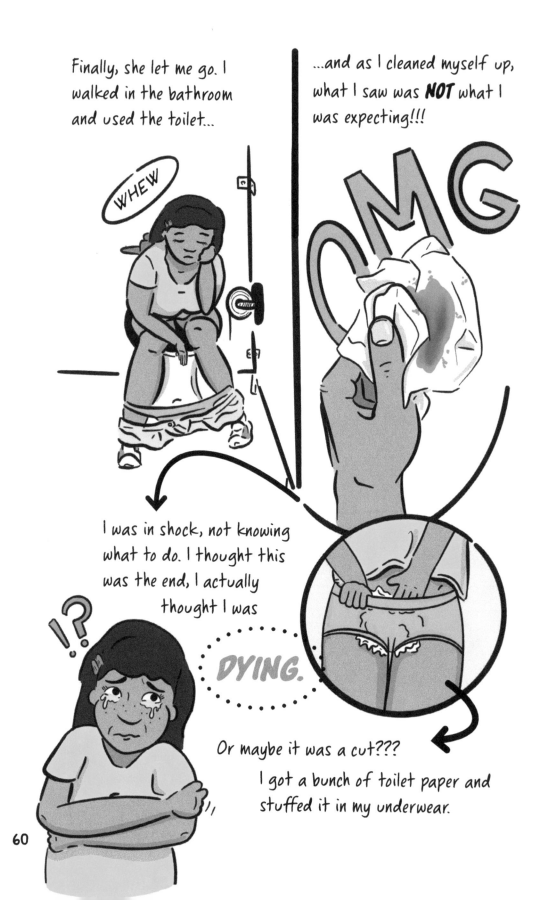

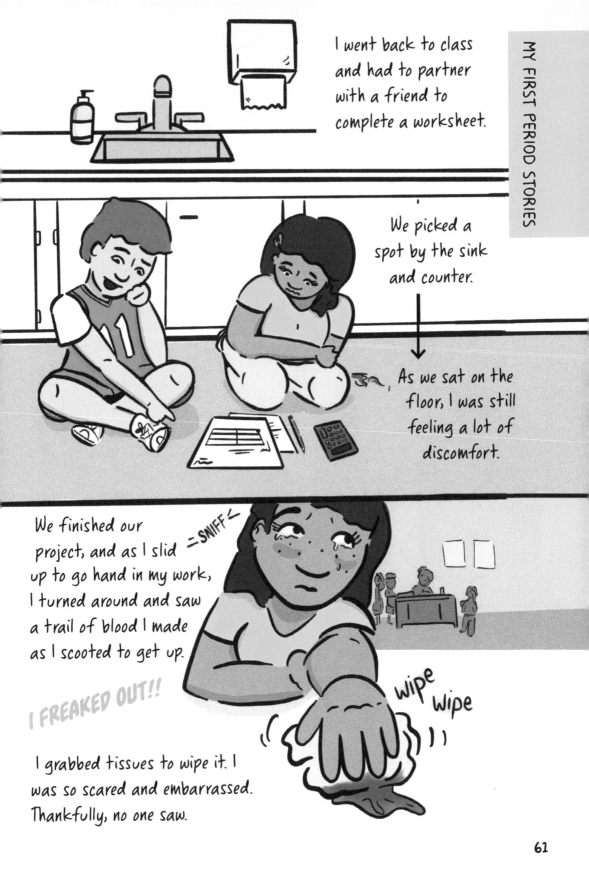

I went back to class and had to partner with a friend to complete a worksheet.

We picked a spot by the sink and counter.

As we sat on the floor, I was still feeling a lot of discomfort.

We finished our project, and as I slid up to go hand in my work, I turned around and saw a trail of blood I made as I scooted to get up.

=SNIFF=

I FREAKED OUT!!

I grabbed tissues to wipe it. I was so scared and embarrassed. Thankfully, no one saw.

wipe wipe

As school ended, I went to my after school program where we would wait for our parents. I was very close to my Aftercare teachers, and I trusted them.

I told them what was happening and that I had to go to the hospital because the bleeding wasn't stopping!!!!

As I told my Aftercare teachers, they started *laughing!*

DON'T WORRY, IT'S OK!

I was **VERY** confused.

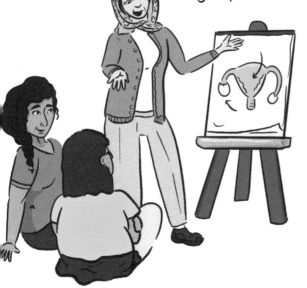

They explained to me what a **PERIOD** is, how it works, and what to do. After that, I felt more educated and realized a whole new chapter of my life had just started.

My teachers came with me to the bathroom, and gave me a pad they had. I used it and felt safer. Then, they called my older brother to pick me up since my clothes were stained.

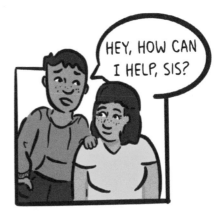

HEY, HOW CAN I HELP, SIS?

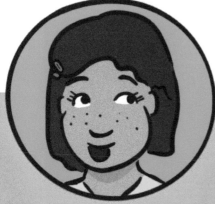

MY ADVICE:

Stay calm and tell a female adult, and they will help you to start your journey. Remember that it's ok if it's irregular or changes schedule sometimes. Bring an extra period product wherever you go! You never know when it may surprise you!

THE END!

STORY 4: MY PURPLE PANTS PANIC

I got my first period while I was at school... and I knew I'd gotten it right as it hit. I was at school in my favorite purple pants and I remember rushing to the bathroom.

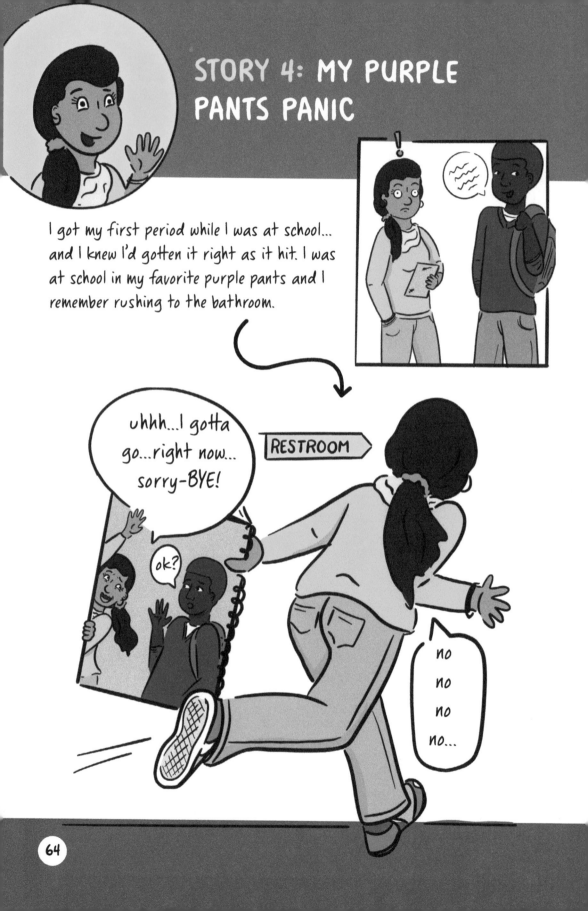

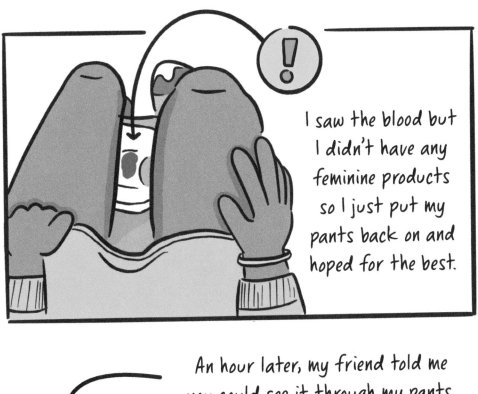

I saw the blood but I didn't have any feminine products so I just put my pants back on and hoped for the best.

An hour later, my friend told me you could see it through my pants.

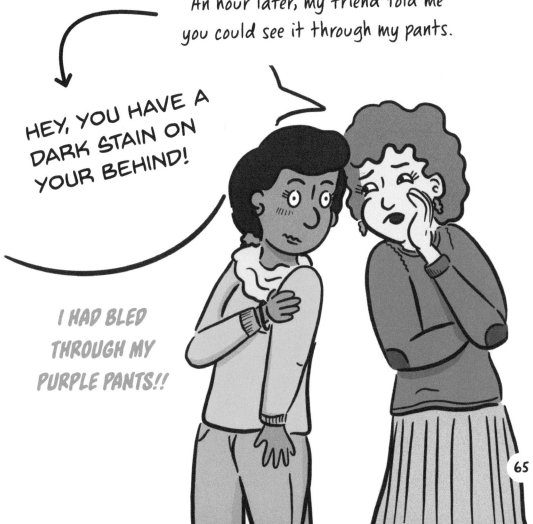

HEY, YOU HAVE A DARK STAIN ON YOUR BEHIND!

I HAD BLED THROUGH MY PURPLE PANTS!!

65

So, I went to the school guidance counselor to hide my pants and sat and talked with her while I waited for my mom to bring me some new pants.

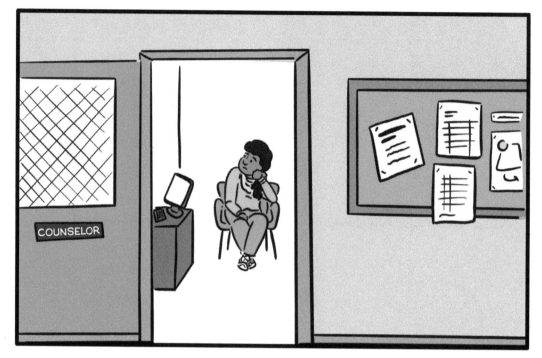

After school, my mom took me to the drug store and taught me the "lay of the land" about pads and tampons.

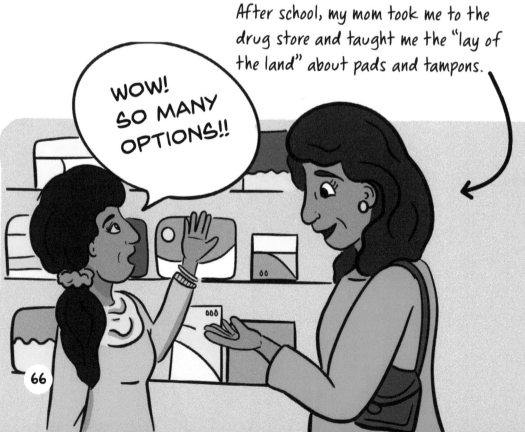

For the remainder of my period, my mom and sister helped me every day to make sure I knew how to change, when to change, and brought me enough supplies.

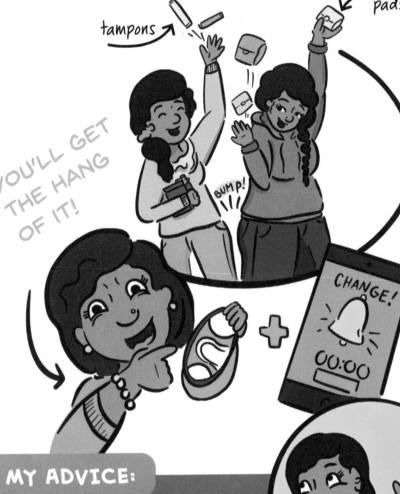

tampons

pads

YOU'LL GET THE HANG OF IT!

BUMP!

CHANGE!

00:00

MY ADVICE:

Don't be scared to get your period, it's perfectly natural. Find an older girl or woman and ask her any and all questions you have. Don't be afraid, we all go through puberty. It's a normal part of growing up!

THE END!

STORY 5: AUNT SARA TO THE RESCUE!!

Well, when I got my first period I was at my aunt's house as my grandmother was out of town.

AUNT SARA'S APARTMENT

MY HOUSE WITH GRANDMA

So it was a Wednesday morning when I woke up, and my lower stomach was hurting REALLY REALLY bad; a kind of pain that I never felt before.

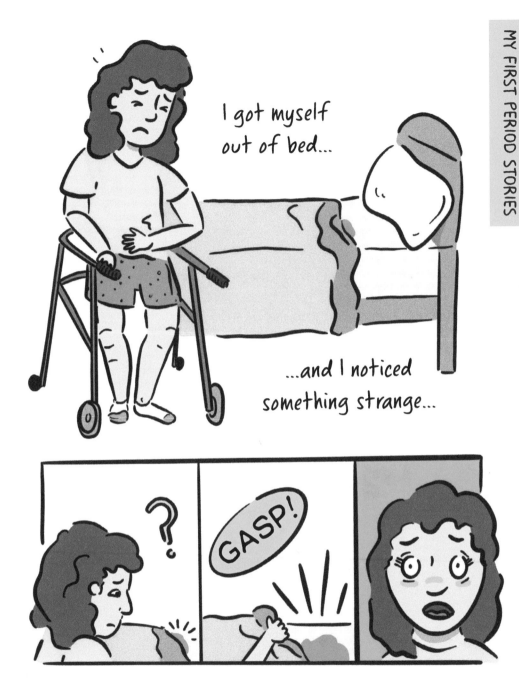

THERE WAS BLOOD
ALL OVER MY SHEETS!

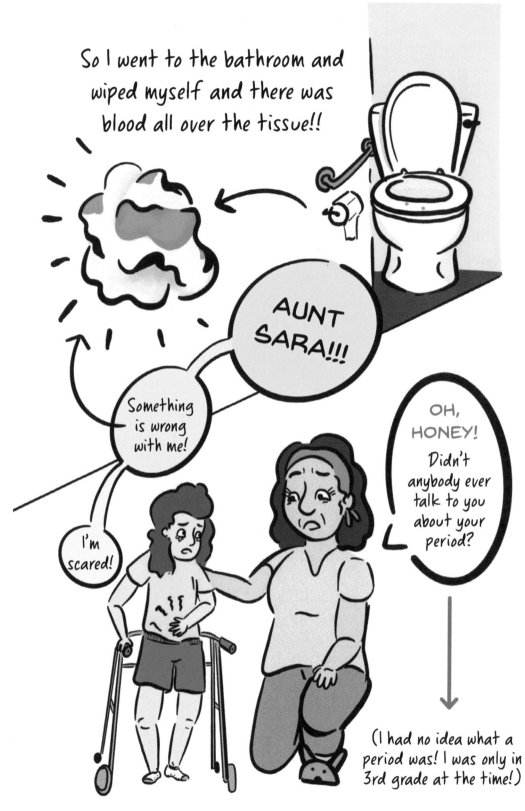

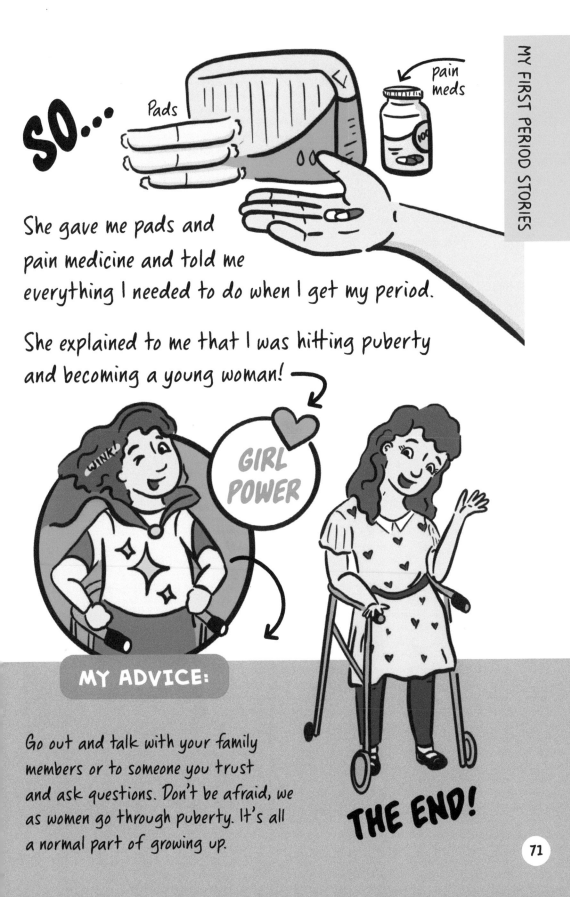

SO...

Pads

pain meds

She gave me pads and pain medicine and told me everything I needed to do when I get my period.

She explained to me that I was hitting puberty and becoming a young woman!

GIRL POWER

WINK!

MY ADVICE:

Go out and talk with your family members or to someone you trust and ask questions. Don't be afraid, we as women go through puberty. It's all a normal part of growing up.

THE END!

71

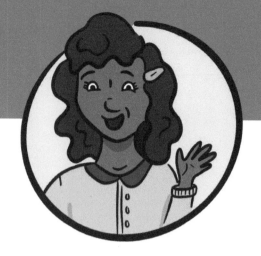

I remember on the day of my first menstrual period, I was in the bathroom at my elementary school.

THE WHOLE DAY I HAD HAD A HEADACHE, AND I FELT A WEIRD FEELING IN MY STOMACH.

Some older girls were huddled around the sink, talking about whether they use 'pads' or 'tampons.' I had no clue what they were talking about.

grumble

They were saying something about blood coming out of their private parts!!

That can't be right, I thought...

I assumed it was bogus but I texted my friend and checked my underwear for blood just in case...and nothing!

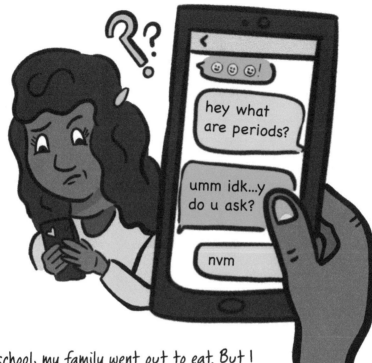

After school, my family went out to eat. But I wasn't feeling well, so we decided to just take our food to go and go home instead.

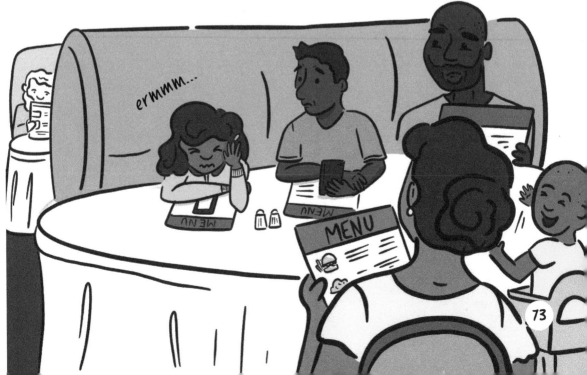

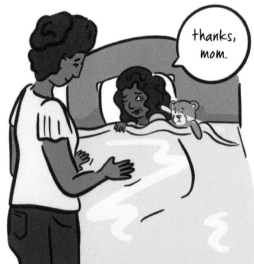

thanks, mom.

I went straight to bed when I got home. It took me a little while to fall asleep, but I finally did, until...

I suddenly woke up, feeling very uncomfortable!!

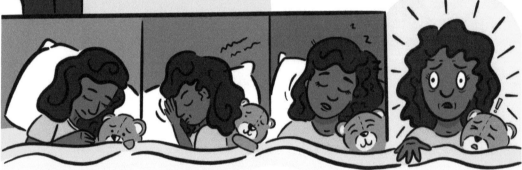

I FELT LIKE I HAD WET THE BED!!

I ran to the bathroom as fast as I could, and as I sat on the toilet, I saw BLOOD in my underwear!!

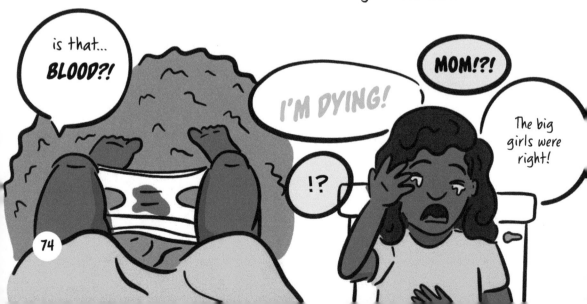

is that... **BLOOD?!**

I'M DYING!

!?

MOM!?!

The big girls were right!

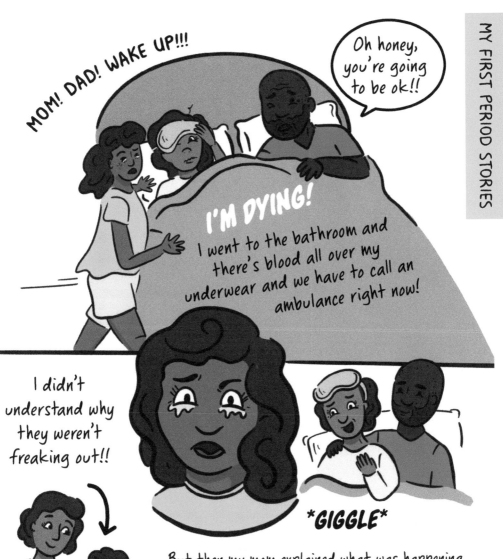

But then my mom explained what was happening and told me how this meant I was a woman. My dad said he knew the day would come where he would have to go to the store and buy his daughter pads.

MY ADVICE:

Try to stay calm, even though it might seem scary, and remember that you aren't alone! Everyone goes through puberty.

THE END!

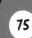

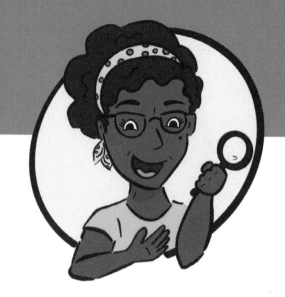

STORY 7: THE CASE OF THE SLOWPOKE PERIOD

My first period came in gradually, for several days near the end of my sixth grade year.

It was really confusing for me at first, and I didn't know what was going on. I didn't understand why there were small brown spots in my underwear.

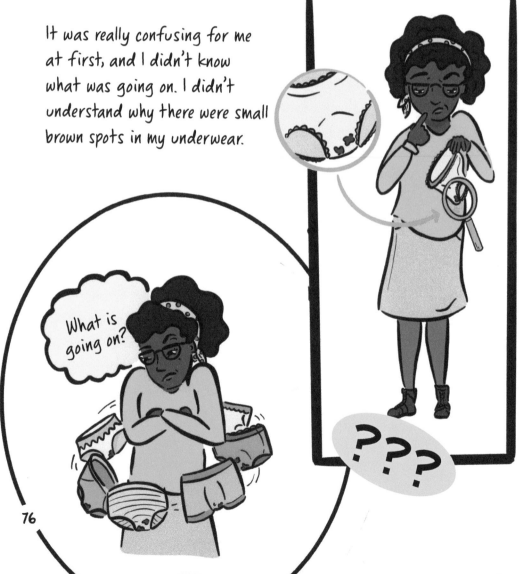

What is going on?

???

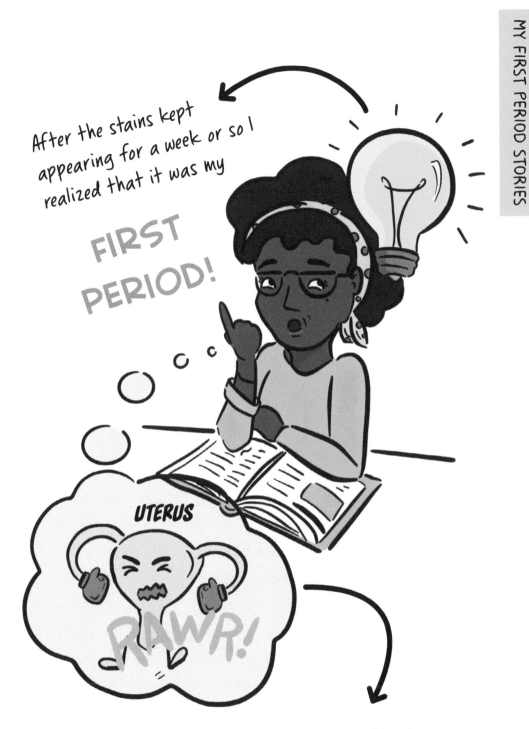

After the stains kept appearing for a week or so I realized that it was my

FIRST PERIOD!

UTERUS

RAWR!

At first I was a bit afraid because I had heard a lot of bad things about <u>menstruation</u>.

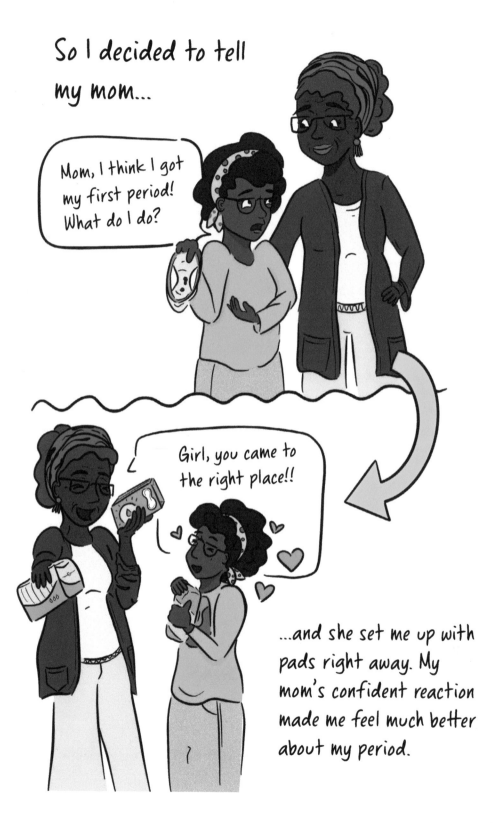

So I decided to tell my mom...

Mom, I think I got my first period! What do I do?

Girl, you came to the right place!!

...and she set me up with pads right away. My mom's confident reaction made me feel much better about my period.

My main fear about <u>menstruation</u> was the cramps, and they aren't fun, but I promise you will survive. There are many ways to reduce the pain from cramping. Find what works best for you!

HEATING PAD

EXERCISE

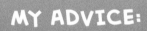

PAIN MEDICINE

The most important thing to remember is that you should not be ashamed of your period or your body and its changes. They are natural, healthy, and there isn't anything wrong with you at all.

MY ADVICE:

Don't be afraid of your period! I understand and agree it can be quite a change, but everything will work itself out.

With time, your period will just become a normal part of your life. **STAY STRONG!**

THE END!

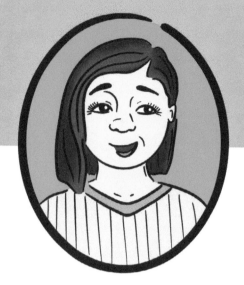

STORY 8: GRANDMA SAVES THE DAY!

I was at my grandma's house when I got my first period. I had a very bad stomach ache which I later learned was <u>CRAMPS</u>.

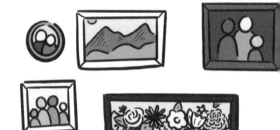

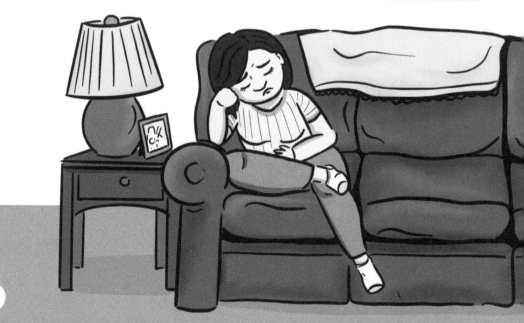

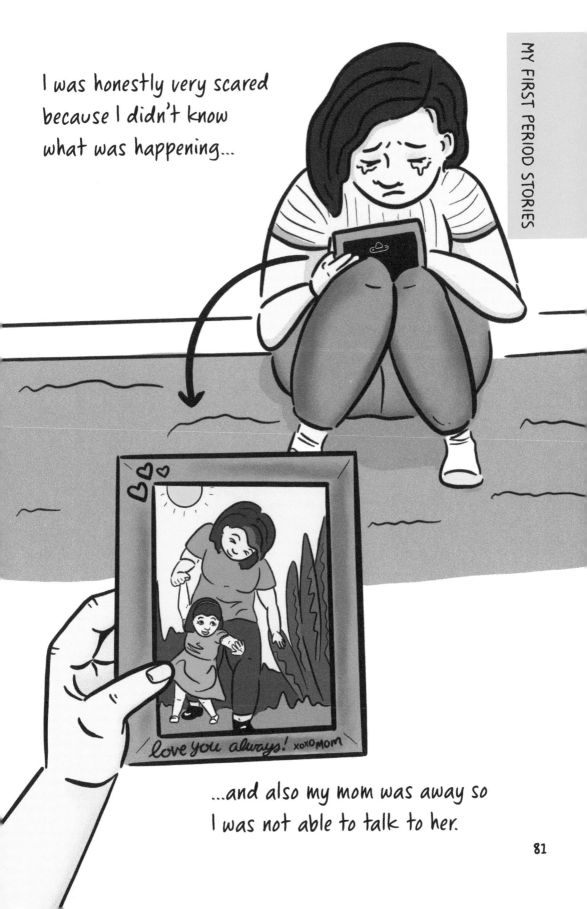

I was honestly very scared because I didn't know what was happening...

love you always! xoxo MOM

...and also my mom was away so I was not able to talk to her.

I didn't tell my grandma because I knew my older cousins had pads in the bathroom.

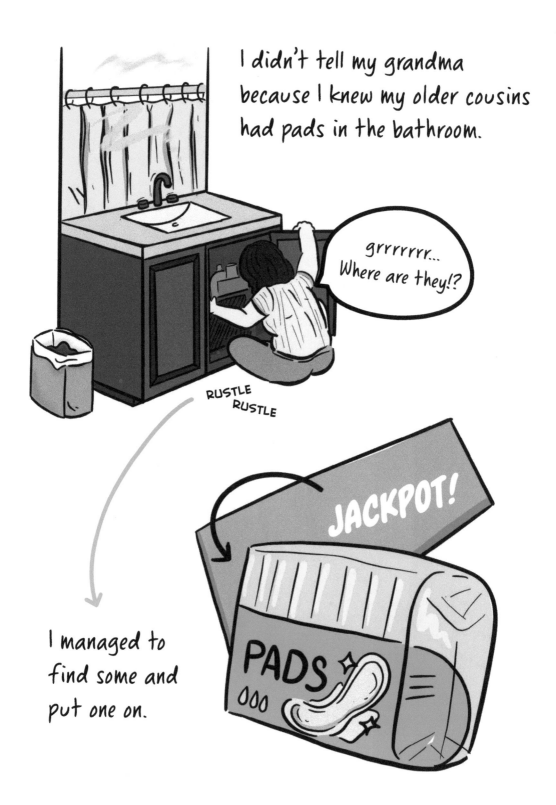

grrrrrrr...
Where are they!?

RUSTLE
RUSTLE

JACKPOT!

PADS

I managed to find some and put one on.

OH NO!!!

When I went home later that night, I realized I did not have any pads or tampons at my house...

GRANDMA

...so I called my grandma because I was scared to tell my dad.

She came by my house and explained everything I needed to know and gave me the supplies I needed for the next week.

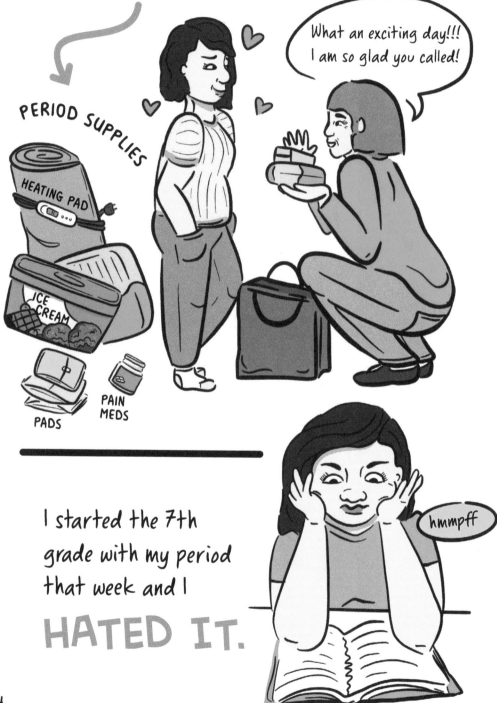

PERIOD SUPPLIES

HEATING PAD

ICE CREAM

PADS

PAIN MEDS

What an exciting day!!! I am so glad you called!

I started the 7th grade with my period that week and I

HATED IT.

hmmpff

Most of my friends helped because they had already gotten their periods so I feel like I got lucky.

I feel like the main thing girls need to know is that they don't need to feel weird or scared to tell someone.

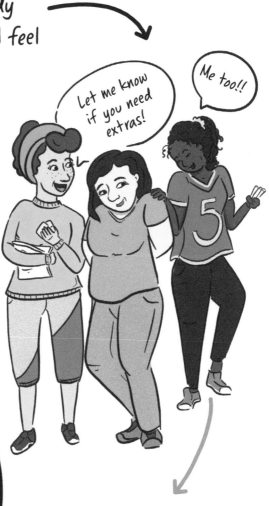

MY ADVICE:

It happens to everyone at a certain point in their life. If you can, find someone you trust and tell them. They will understand and they will help you.

THE END!

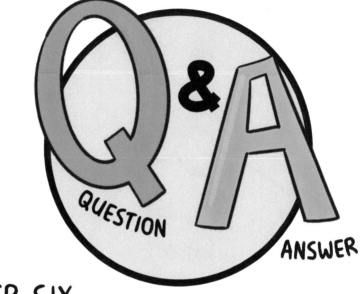

CHAPTER SIX
ALL THE FACTS!

PERIOD MYTH BUSTERS!

We often hear lots of advice and ideas about periods. Some of it is true and some of it is not.

Can you tell which ones are TRUE OR FALSE?

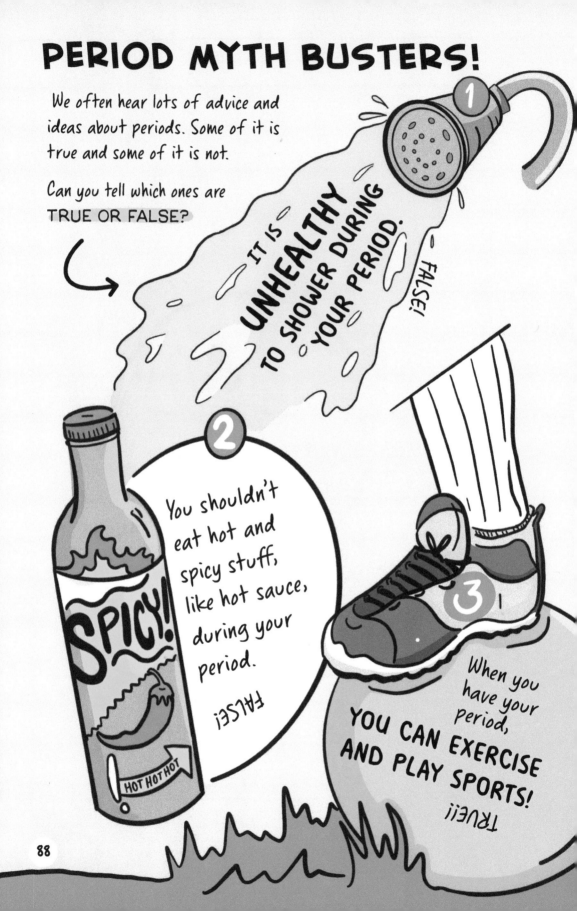

1 IT IS UNHEALTHY TO SHOWER DURING YOUR PERIOD. — FALSE!

2 You shouldn't eat hot and spicy stuff, like hot sauce, during your period. FALSE!

SPICY!! HOT HOT HOT

3 When you have your period, YOU CAN EXERCISE AND PLAY SPORTS! TRUE!!

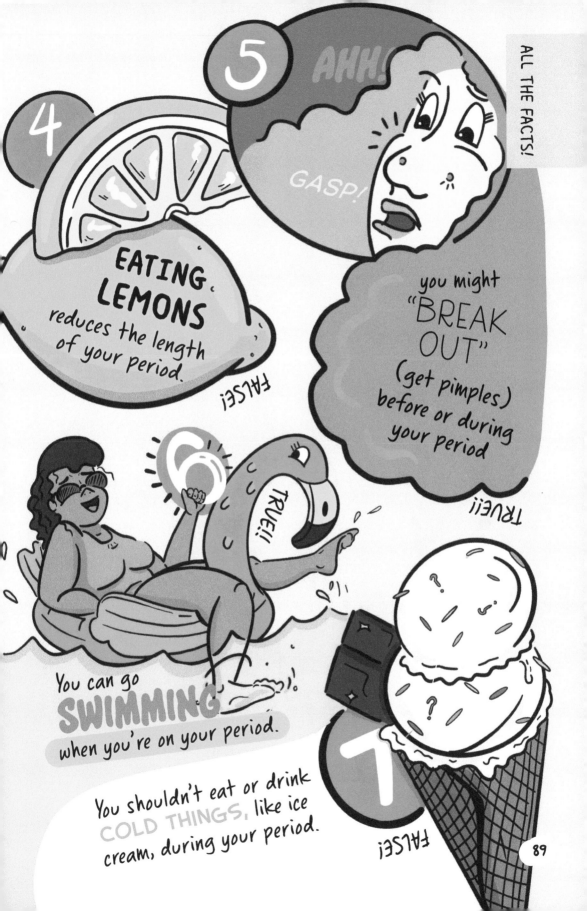

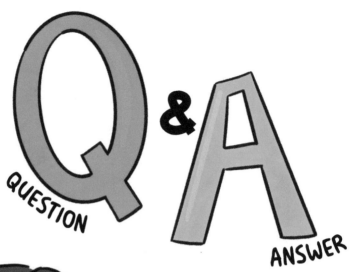

Q & A

QUESTION | ANSWER

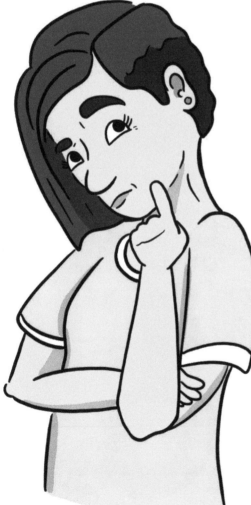

It's normal to have A LOT of questions! Here are some answers to common questions girls have about body changes and periods.

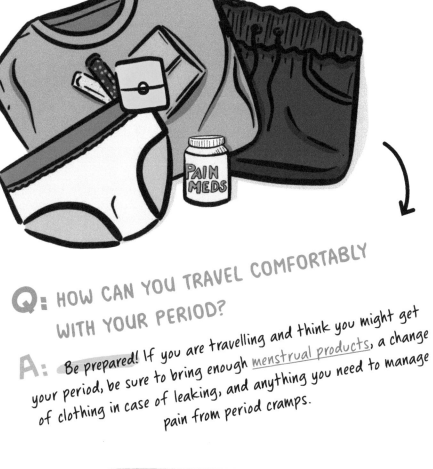

Q: HOW CAN YOU TRAVEL COMFORTABLY WITH YOUR PERIOD?

A: Be prepared! If you are travelling and think you might get your period, be sure to bring enough <u>menstrual products</u>, a change of clothing in case of leaking, and anything you need to manage pain from period cramps.

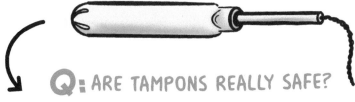

Q: ARE TAMPONS REALLY SAFE?

A: Tampons are inserted into the vagina during menstruation in order to absorb menstrual flow. They are very safe to use, as long as you change them every 6-8 hours or more often. It can be helpful to read the instructions found on the product box. Don't worry, they can't get lost in your vagina. There are many menstrual products available though, and you get to decide what you want to use. Some families aren't comfortable with tampons, so if you're unsure, talk to them about it.

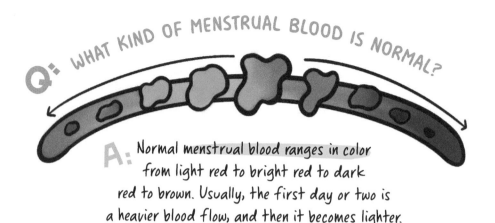

Q: WHAT KIND OF MENSTRUAL BLOOD IS NORMAL?

A: Normal menstrual blood ranges in color from light red to bright red to dark red to brown. Usually, the first day or two is a heavier blood flow, and then it becomes lighter.

Q: WHAT DOES IT MEAN IF YOU HAVE BLOOD CLOTS IN YOUR PERIOD BLOOD?

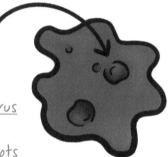

A: It's perfectly normal! The lining of the uterus that sheds during menstruation is made up of blood and tissue, so it is common to see small clots or clumps of blood during your period.

Q: WHAT IS THE WHITE GOOEY STUFF THAT CAN BE IN YOUR UNDERWEAR SOMETIMES?

A: The white stuff is called vaginal discharge. It is totally normal and nothing to be embarrassed about. Normal discharge (clear, white, off white) is healthy. If the discharge becomes very thick with a chunky-like texture or fishy smell that could be a sign of an infection, so you may want to visit a medical professional or talk to an adult you trust just to be safe.

Q: AT WHAT AGE IS IT NORMAL TO GET YOUR FIRST PERIOD?

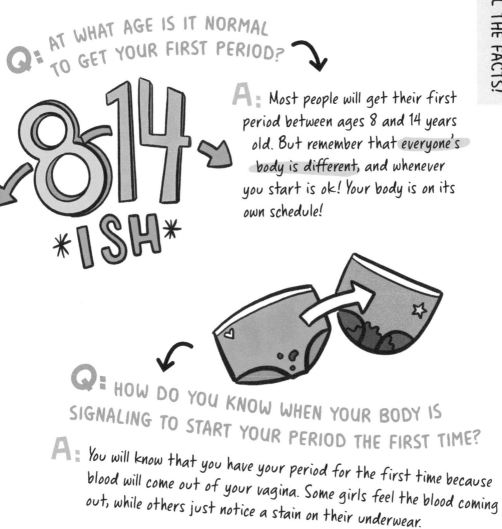

A: Most people will get their first period between ages 8 and 14 years old. But remember that everyone's body is different, and whenever you start is ok! Your body is on its own schedule!

Q: HOW DO YOU KNOW WHEN YOUR BODY IS SIGNALING TO START YOUR PERIOD THE FIRST TIME?

A: You will know that you have your period for the first time because blood will come out of your vagina. Some girls feel the blood coming out, while others just notice a stain on their underwear.

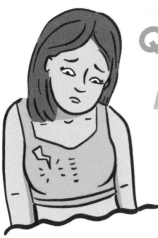

Q: IS IT NATURAL TO GET SOME BREAST PAINS?

A: Yes, many people will experience breast tenderness, especially right before or during their period. Your breasts may also feel a little sore sometimes as part of the growing process.

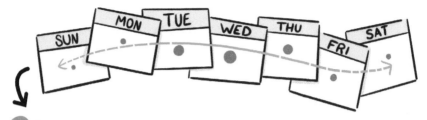

Q: WHY IS MY PERIOD SOMETIMES ONLY 3 DAYS AND SOMETIMES AS LONG AS 7 DAYS?

A: Everyone's cycle length is different, and yours may change over time. For the first year or two after you start your period, it's normal to be irregular. It will likely become more regular over time.

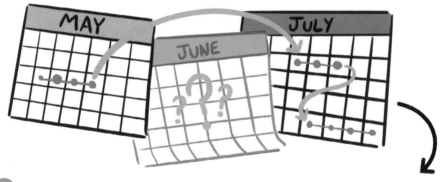

Q: WHY DOES MY PERIOD SKIP SOMETIMES? AND/ OR OCCUR MORE THAN ONE TIME PER MONTH?

A: For a year or two after you start your period, it's normal for your cycle to be irregular, but it will likely become more regular over time. Your period doesn't go by the "month" exactly. It happens on average every 25 — 35 days. So that may mean you get it twice in one "month"!

WHY DO SOME GIRLS GET CRAMPS AND SOME DON'T?

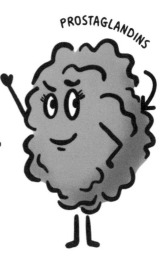

PROSTAGLANDINS

A: It all depends on the hormones in your body! Hormones called "prostaglandins" help the uterus shed its lining during your period, and they also cause menstrual cramps. Some people have more prostaglandins than others, and so they might experience more severe menstrual cramps.

Q: WHAT CAN HELP CRAMPS BESIDES MEDICATION?

A: Using a heating pad, sitting in a hot bath, or getting some exercise can make cramps feel better. If this doesn't help, talk to a parent, doctor, or another adult you trust about your cramps.

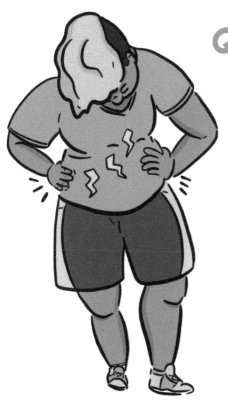

Q: ARE EXTREMELY PAINFUL CRAMPS NORMAL?

A: Some period cramps are normal, but they shouldn't keep you from playing sports, going to school, or doing any of your regular activities. If your cramps are so painful that you aren't able to go about your day normally, you should talk to a doctor or a trusted adult.

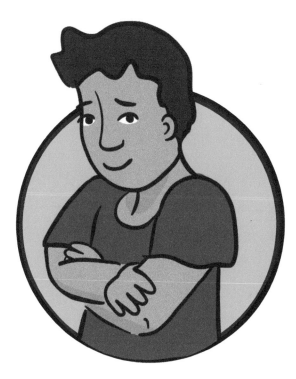

CHAPTER SEVEN
WHAT ABOUT BOYS?

SO WHAT'S GOING ON IN
HIS BODY??

Boys also have so many changes in their bodies during puberty! Some of these changes are physical, some are emotional, and some are the same as girls!

They grow taller and gain weight too. They get hair in new places, like their <u>pubic</u> area, under their arms and on their faces! Their bodies also become more oily, so they can also get pimples and new body smells.

MUSCLE GROWTH

GETTING TALLER!!

FACIAL HAIR & PIMPLES TOO!

Boys also experience changes in their emotions, including feeling highs and lows.

SO WHAT'S
DIFFERENT FOR BOYS?

Well, they don't get periods!

Their bodies are built differently and inside their organs and hormones are different. They get facial hair, bigger muscles, and their voices change!

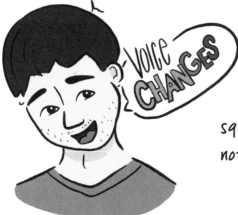

VOICE CHANGES

It can be embarrassing for them when their voices squeak as they change, so try not to laugh!

Boys also get something called nocturnal emissions (or "wet dreams"), and something called erections, which is when the penis fills with blood and becomes harder.

It can be embarrassing or uncomfortable for a boy to get used to these changes. They can't control them any more than a girl can control a period.

99

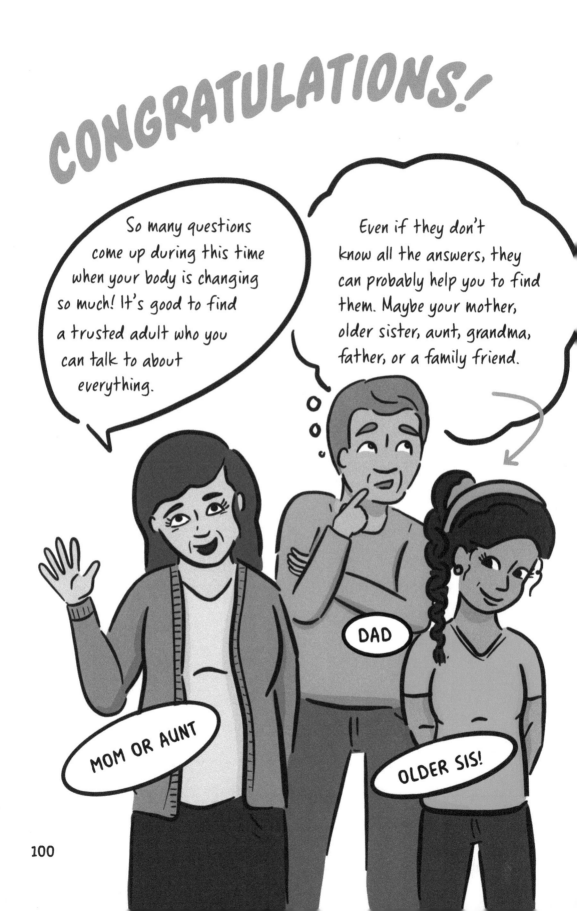

You are going through such an exciting time of change, with so much changing inside and outside your body.

FEEL PROUD AND CONFIDENT ABOUT YOUR BODY CHANGES!

They are special to you, and it's all a part of growing up!

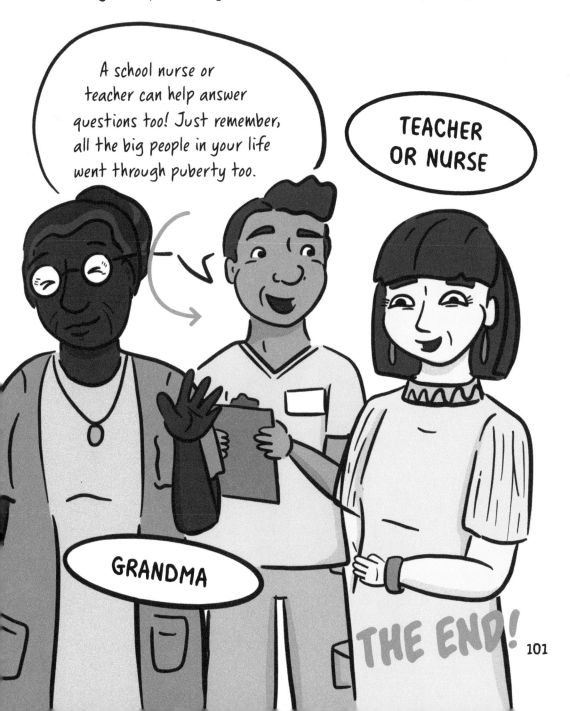

A school nurse or teacher can help answer questions too! Just remember, all the big people in your life went through puberty too.

TEACHER OR NURSE

GRANDMA

THE END!

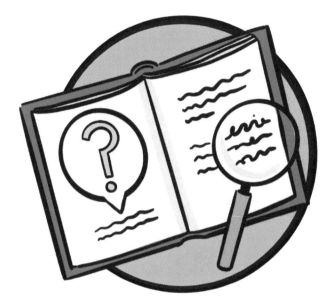

GLOSSARY

GLOSSARY

AREOLAS

Areolas (air-ee-oh-luhs) are the darker, round area around the nipples on your breasts. They range in color (from pink to red to brown to black) and size.

BLOATING

Bloating is a symptom that many people experience before and during their period. It might feel like your belly is swollen or very full.

CLOTS/CLUMPS

As the uterus sheds its lining, it's normal to have gel-like blobs or clumps of blood or tissue (also known as "clots") that come out of the vagina during menstruation.

EGGS

Eggs are one of the sex cells needed to start a pregnancy.

ESTROGEN AND PROGESTERONE

Estrogen (eh-struh-jn) and Progesterone (pro-jeh-str-own) are hormones that are important for body development during puberty, mainly in girls.

MENSTRUAL PRODUCTS

Menstrual products, such as pads and tampons, are items used during a period to absorb menstrual blood.

MENSTRUATION

Menstruation (men-stroo-A-shun) is another word for having a period. Menstruation is when the uterus sheds blood and tissue out of the vagina, usually for a few days every month after puberty starts. This is also called a menstrual cycle.

OVULATION

Ovulation (ah-vyuh-lay-shun) is when an egg is released from an ovary, which usually happens about once every month after puberty starts.

PREMENSTRUAL SYNDROME

Premenstrual Syndrome (pree-men-struhl) (sin-drowm) or PMS describes the emotional changes, or "mood swings" that can fluctuate with someone's menstrual cycle. It can also include other symptoms like breast tenderness, food cravings, bloating, back pain, and tiredness.

PROSTAGLANDINS

Prostaglandins (pra-sta-glan-dinz) are hormones that help the uterus squeeze out the blood and tissue during menstruation. When the uterus squeezes, some people feel cramps in their lower belly or back area.

PUBIC

Pubic (pyoo-bic) is the triangular area just above the vagina and below the belly. People start to grow hair around their pubic area during puberty.